A
HOSPITAL
HANDBOOK
ON
MULTICULTURALISM
AND RELIGION

NEVILLE A. KIRKWOOD

First published in 1993 by
Millennium Books, an imprint of
E. J. Dwyer (Australia) Pty Ltd
3/32-72 Alice Street
Newtown NSW 2042
Australia
Phone: (02) 550-2355
Fax: (02) 519-3218

National Library of Australia
Cataloguing-in-Publication data

Kirkwood, Neville A. (Neville Allan), 1927–   .
   A hospital handbook on multiculturalism and religion.

   Bibliography.
   ISBN 0 85574 921 0.

   1. Minorities—Medical care—Australia. 2. Hospital patients—
   Australia—Social conditions. 3. Medicine—Religious aspects. 4.
   Social medicine—Australia. 5. Pluralism (Social sciences)—
   Australia. 6. Religions. I. Title.

362.108693

Cover design by Luc Oechslin, Tatum Graphics, Sydney.
Text design by Katrina Rendell.
Typeset in 10½/12pt Cheltenham Light by Post Typesetters, Qld.
Printed in Australia by Griffin Paperbacks, Adelaide

About the author

Neville Kirkwood is well experienced in relating to cultural groups and in hospital protocol, having been a fulltime hospital chaplain for sixteen years. After tertiary studies in theology at the Queensland Baptist College and the Melbourne College of Divinity, Neville earned the Doctorate of Ministry through the San Francisco Theological Seminary. He has recently been the President of The Australian College of Chaplains.

Acknowledgements

The following organisations are hereby acknowledged for their helpful responses to my enquiries and for their publications:

- The Maronite Church (Sydney diocese)
- The Syrian Orthodox Church of Antioch
- The Greek Orthodox Archdiocese of Australia
- The Church of Christ Theological College, Sydney
- The Salvation Army
- The Seventh-Day Adventist Church
- The Roman Catholic Church (Sydney archdiocese)
- The Baptist Union of N.S.W.
- The Anglican Church (Sydney archdiocese)
- The Church of Jesus Christ of Latter-Day Saints
- The National Spiritual Assembly of the Bahá'ís
- The Lothian Community Relations Council, Edinburgh
- The Australian Buddhist Vihara Institute
- The Buddhist Society of N.S.W.
- The Presbyterian Church of Australia
- The Islamic Council of N.S.W.
- The N.S.W. Jewish Board of Deputies
- The Lisa Sainsbury Foundation, London
- The Hospital Chaplaincies Council, London
- Ms. Pamela Bennet, Japan
- *Nursing Times*, Macmillan Publishing, London

Foreword

Australia is now the most multicultural nation in the world. This diversity of peoples of different cultures and religions offers an important challenge for health services committed to the provision of care and services which are appropriate and accessible and which recognise and value people's different cultural and religious backgrounds.

An individual's culture and religion form fundamental parts of their make-up and are particularly important when that person is seriously ill and in hospital. It is recognised that different cultural behaviours and religious beliefs can lead to misunderstandings between health professionals and the people in their care. It is therefore important for staff to be sensitive to the particular attitudes and needs of their patients and of the relatives of those patients.

Reverend Dr. Kirkwood's hospital handbook

represents a commendable effort to provide accessible information on this diverse and complex topic and is a valuable addition to our growing knowledge about the needs of our multicultural society. It provides insight into the different beliefs and practices of the major religions, as well as discussing the significance of certain religious attitudes and rites to the lives of the people of these religions. It also includes information on what action may be taken by lay persons in some emergency situations, action that may bring comfort and peace of mind to those concerned.

I believe that if used to complement information gained directly from patients and professionals it will prove most useful for the continuing development of appropriate and sensitive health care for people here and elsewhere.

B. J. AMOS
Director-General
N.S.W. Department of Health
Sydney
Australia

Contents

Introduction

Many health care workers, including chaplains, are unfamiliar with multicultural needs and requirements. This handbook is intended to be a ready-reference for those who work in hospitals and similar institutions dealing with the sick.

The last half of the twentieth century has seen distance become of minimal consequence in our world. The movement of peoples from country to country either as tourists, refugees or in migration has escalated in recent decades.

It started with the population shifts following World War II. Independence from colonial powers saw many nationals of their former colonies taking advantage of concessions granted by the former rulers. And there was also the resettlement of post-war displaced people from Europe.

More recently the wars in Indo-China and the Middle East, particularly Lebanon, have resulted in the considerable re-settlement of the victims of these wars. Indo-China, with its many differing cultures, has added new dimensions to Australia's multicultural mix. The Middle East situation has enabled Islam to be more widely recognised here where previously it was comparatively unknown.

The developing of the economy of Korea, Hong Kong and Japan has spread their people abroad. Their appearance in Western society (either as migrants, business people or tourists) means that they are being met in our hospitals and health care institutions. As the Japanese culture involves an intermingling of practices, there is a final chapter, "Japanese beliefs and practices", to enhance understanding in this area.

As I said at the beginning, this book is intended for reference. However, in any country where cultures intermingle, the practices of a particular culture, which includes its religious aspects, are likely to be modified or adapted to the parameters of the local environment. Thus this is a handbook providing guidelines which should not be used as a substitute for or to avoid face-to-face assessment of the patient's own religious views and practices. Rather it should be used, as Dr. Amos suggests in his Foreword, to supplement information coming directly from the patient and family and only used as the first source of information where this information is not directly available from the patient or family themselves.

* * *

With regard to Australian Aborigines, where they constitute a large percentage of hospital admissions, particularly beyond the coastal fringe, hospitals have already developed procedures in catering for their needs. In some areas, they have their own Aboriginal Health Services. Hospitals are always able to consult the Aboriginal and Torres Strait Islander Commission in their region for information on the requirements of Aboriginal patients.

1. A multicultural society

The debate over multiculturalism and integration or assimilation has been—and sometimes still is—a minefield of insensitivity on both sides. Host cultures are often intolerant of the differences which peoples of other cultures bring. The newcomers expect their hosts to permit them to live and function as they would in their native land. Differences in the standard and style of living are often ignored.

A move from a third world country to the West brings such a contrast that sometimes the adjustment is made even more difficult. A need to maintain cultural practices is necessary for the stability of the newcomer in a strange land. The desire to live close to fellow countrymen, which establishes cultural enclaves, is natural. Yet this very process is often misunderstood. People grieving for a homeland need support both from fellow countrymen and the citizens of their adopted country.

The one area where all must be treated on equal terms is in the health care field. Health care workers have a reputation for being caring, understanding people. Because of this, they are aware that these newcomers have different beliefs and customs which need to be considered in the hospital setting. Different religious traditions have led to certain practices and behaviour. These need to be respected, particularly when and where there is a person dying. Respect for these requirements is essential for the healthy grief of the relatives and friends. The staff also need to be comfortable in the knowledge that what they have done is acceptable.

It is easy for our Western psychology-trained hospital bereavement counsellor to be alarmed, for instance, that a certain group of a particular ethnic origin are apparently showing no sign of grief or are not talking about the imminent death of their family patriarch. It may be the practice in these people's culture for the second degree male relatives (e.g. uncles or cousins) to be the ones with whom the doctors and staff discuss the nature of the patient's diagnosis and response to treatment. The second degree relatives then decide who and how much should be told. Often the nuclear family of the relative is unaware of the seriousness of the illness.

People from such a background fear to mention the possibility of a terminal condition. For them to name a condition is to open the possibility for its fulfilment. For social workers, chaplains, nurses or doctors to raise the question of possible death, without first endeavouring to understand the cultural stance, is likely to cause the family bewilderment and confusion. There may even be a communication breakdown between the medical team and the patient's kin.

To assume that because patients are in a Western hospital they can shed millennia of cultural inheritance to conform with different cultural perspectives is to misunderstand the value of cultural practice. For some it may adversely affect the progress or response to treatment. It is not a case of either assimilation or multiculturalism. There needs to be a marriage of the two. The staff and patient each must seek to learn from each other, each being prepared to not only live as neighbours but also to respect areas of habit or cultural emphasis in the interests of harmonious co-operation.

Within health care institutions socio-religious concerns are of great importance, no matter the country of origin or religion of the people involved. Of course, there are always some who are devout in their religious practice and others who are indifferent.

Due deference should be given to the socio-religious requirements of hospital patients, particularly in a time of crisis. Offers of assistance to seek out the appropriate religious person for the patient in no way must be given the appearance of interference or cause embarrassment to the patient. The priest of the patient's faith should be notified.

In hospitals where there are numbers of patients of different ethnic backgrounds, staff should make some effort to be aware of these differences. In each religion there are groups with different emphases or differing sects or denominations, as found within the Christian religion. It is not possible for each health care worker to be able to identify all these divisions. With a sense of caring, the particular persuasion or preference of the patient may be ascertained either from the patient or the relatives.

There may be members of staff who belong to the same faith, whether they are domestic, catering or ward staff. If a professional interpreter is not available they may be requested to ascertain the religious position of the patient and identify the patient's significant adviser, priest, imam or rabbi. There may be other appropriate ways of discovering the desired information, but if there are language problems, using an experienced interpreter is the ideal solution.

It cannot be over-emphasised that not only may people from other backgrounds have practices and beliefs which differ from Western Christianity, but it must be understood that religious traditions are part of culture. The culture of an Asian Christian may therefore differ from the cultural practices of a Greek or Dutch Christian. There are cultural distinctions as well as specifically-religious variations to daily living: so that a Vietnamese Christian, for instance, will have customs and beliefs that will differ from those of a Vietnamese Buddhist. Similarly a Vietnamese Christian will have needs which may not be entirely akin to an Australian-born Christian's requirements; and, further, a Roman Catholic patient will desire certain sacraments to be administered whilst a Baptist may not be so insistent, though all are Christians.

When it comes to hospital bedside treatment and procedures during hospitalisation or at death, there are certain questions which should be considered as far as possible by the staff. These involve diet, fasting, names, symbols, birth, and handling of the body on death. Some of these basic matters will be outlined in the following pages.

Integration or Westernisation to varying degrees

depending upon the patient's age, education and cultural roots must be expected. The health care worker must be alert to discern to what degree the ways of the country of adoption have been adsorbed by the patient and family members. This can vary from person to person and within a family. The patriarch or matriarch of a family may be a key to the amount of assimilation that has taken place. He or she may be so revered as to be able to enforce within the family the strict observance of cultural traditions.

On the other hand, for example, a Hindu patient who in his own country was a strict vegetarian, may readily eat meat, even beef, in his new land.

Each patient and family needs to have some sort of assessment made as to how strictly they observe their culture and religion. This may be done at the initial admission by a questionnaire which includes matters of diet, religious persons to contact, fasting or other specific needs, such as special arrangements when using the toilet. (Many people from the East prefer water cleansing rather than the use of toilet paper.)

The following chapters will deal with each religion or culture separately. These should be used as background information and as a guide. They should not be used as a substitute for the opportunity to talk with a patient or family about their religion and culture. Most respond to sincere enquiries about their beliefs and practices. Their awareness of your interest breaks down fears and worry about being misunderstood. It opens the way for mutual appreciation and co-operation within the ward. This in turn makes for a patient who is more ready to accept the necessary treatment and hospitalisation in a strange environment.

2. Christianity

In the Western world, Christianity has dominated history, religion, politics, law and education for centuries. In the last half of the twentieth century humanism, secularism, materialism, more recently the "new age" movement and the influence of Marxism and neomarxism has seen a decline in the awareness and practice of Christianity. Basic Biblical knowledge, its meaning and application are not as widespread nor are the practices of the various denominations of the Christian church so well known, some of which have undergone reform. In looking at a Christian's needs we shall consider them under five major groupings, noting any particular variations in practice. They are Catholics, Orthodox, Established churches, Non-conformists and others, a more or less historical division.

(a) *Catholics:* Roman, Maronite, Jacobite, Melchite, and Ukrainian.

(b) *Orthodox:* Eastern (Russian and Greek), Syrian, Serbian, Coptic, Armenian, Lebanese, Bulgarian, Polish, and Macedonian.

(c) *Established churches* (i.e. those churches which were recognised and established as the church of the state): Anglican (Church of England, Episcopal), Lutheran, Church of Scotland, Reformed Dutch.

(d) *Non-conformist, Independent* (those churches which separated from the established churches): Baptist, Church of Christ, Congregational, Methodist, Presbyterian, Salvation Army, Seventh-Day Adventist, Uniting Church, Pentecostal and neo-Pentecostal.

(e) *Others:* Church of the Latter-Day Saints (Mormons), Jehovah's Witnesses.

The Catholic, Orthodox and some established churches have an episcopal form of church government, that is, a system of bishops. They place a stronger emphasis on the position and status of the clergy. Generally the priest's principal ministry is the administration of the sacraments. For many of their parishioners who are patients in a hospital, receiving the sacraments is important in a religious sense, as well as having therapeutic benefit.

For non-conformists and some others, the ministry of the sacraments plays an important but less central role in worship and life of the church. The ministry of the word, Biblical teaching and pastoral care (other than the sacramental) have the greater emphasis.

Christians believe that Jesus, born about 6 BC in Bethlehem in Judea, was the messiah, or Christ, promised through the previous millennia through the Hebrews to the world by their God, Yahweh. This messiah was to be God in human form. This Jesus is God from eternity. The death experienced by Jesus was the means of atonement whereby men and women may experience the forgiveness of God and be restored into a personal relationship with him.

True Christianity is not knowledge or belief in a set of historical events; rather it is the acceptance of those historical events as God acting to draw humankind to himself in unique intimacy. It is a spiritual communion between God and the believer. Through this relationship, God's way of love and peace should be demonstrated to the historical world.

Christian pastoral care in the hospital setting is carried out in the name of Christ. The integrity of the Christian carer may be sufficient testimony of the Christian nature of the care offered. At other times it is appropriate to counsel or to share the Christian way in the course of the caring or to provide Christian spiritual support and comfort through scripture reading, sacrament, prayer and other means.

I. RITUALS AND SACRAMENTS

Most religions have set rituals and sacraments. Christian denominations variously celebrate the major events in a person's life such as birth, marriage and death. There are also other sacraments which hold spiritual significance, such as confession (reconciliation), anointings and the Eucharist (holy communion) which may be important for many hospitalised people.

(a) Catholic Group

A visit from a chaplain or priest is considered normal practice. Such a visit will ascertain the patient's need for the sacraments. Any request for a chaplain or priest should be treated as of utmost importance. Catholics believe the spiritual needs should be given higher priority than the physical and temporal.

The chaplain or priests are able to provide more than sacramental ministry; counsel and emotional support are roles which they willingly accept with the patients or relatives.

Baptism

This sacrament brings to a person a share in the life of Christ and membership of his church.

Where a baby or unbaptised Catholic person's life is in danger, the chaplain or priest should be called. In an emergency, if a chaplain or priest is not available, any person may baptise. In such cases the baptising person pours water on the child and says the words: "I baptise you in the name of the Father and of the Son and of the Holy Spirit". When an emergency baptism is conferred, the chaplain or priest is to be notified later, so that details may be registered.

Reconciliation (Confession)

This sacrament brings to the Catholic in a particular way a loving God's reassurance. The sacrament can be given only by a priest. Privacy is essential.

Holy communion

Catholics believe that Jesus is present in this special sacrament and therefore the communicant is united with Christ in a special way. The sacrament of Holy Communion may be administered by a priest or a person who has the endorsement of the chaplain. The chaplain or priest will consult staff in deciding whether holy communion can be given to a patient (who may be nauseated or fasting before an anaesthetic) who may gave requested it. Where necessary, patients can be given a particle so small that it will not interfere with medical or surgical procedures.

Anointing of the sick

In this sacrament patients are offered the compassion of Jesus for the sick, it gives them strength and peace. It is given only by a priest. A patient may be anointed more than once during the same illness. Catholics have an expectation that a priest will be called in a case of emergency and this should be done when a known Catholic lapses into unconsciousness or is unable to communicate his or her wishes. This sacrament is not given to a person who has died; therefore a chaplain or priest should be called before death occurs.

A sacramental ministry by a Roman Catholic priest is acceptable to patients of the other Catholic churches identified here, when a priest of their own church is unavailable.

(b) Orthodox Group

Baptism

If a new born babe's condition warrants serious concern for its survival, a priest should be contacted, with the parent's consent, for the sacrament of holy baptism.

If an orthodox priest is not available, any Christian priest or minister may perform an emergency baptism by raising the child in the air and saying: "The servant of God (name) is baptised in the name of the Father and of the Son and of the Holy Spirit. Amen". If the lifting of the child is not possible, then baptism may be administered by placing the right hand on the bowl of water which should be available. The Orthodox priest should be informed of such emergency baptisms.

Confession
When requested by the patient, the priest should be called. Privacy for total confidentiality should of course be provided if possible.

Holy communion
This may be received as often as possible for spiritual and bodily sanctification. Patients scheduled for an operation should receive holy communion the day before if possible. Holy communion given at such time is not equivalent to last rites. Baptism precludes the necessity for last rites for the Greek Orthodox patient.

Last anointing
The Syrian Orthodox priest administers the sacrament of the last anointing. Usually it is administered before death, but may be dispensed after the patient's apparent death in the hope that the Spirit is still in the body. Prior to this anointing, confession and holy communion should be offered if possible.

(c) Established Group
Baptism
In an emergency, a staff member such as a nurse may pour a little water on the baby's head saying: "(Name) I baptise you in the name of the Father and

of the Son and of the Holy Spirit". When there is time, the chaplain or clergyman should be called. The one officiating would desire (if possible) to meet the parents before conducting the baptism. Certificates of baptism should be issued. If the baby survives, the parents should contact the Parish minister to complete the service.

Holy communion
This is celebrated by a fully-ordained clergyperson. Communication is usually provided on the request of the patient or relatives. It is desirable, when possible, that more than one person with the minister celebrate holy communion.

Last anointing
There are no last rites. Prayers and the offer of comfort and support are given by the church to the family at the time of death, on the request of relatives.

(d) Non-conformist or Independent

The Salvation Army do not observe any sacraments such as baptism or holy communion.

Baptism
Baptists, Church of Christ, Seventh-Day Adventist and some Pentecostals and Neo-Pentecostals followers practice believers' baptism. This service is conducted only after the individual has reached an age where an understanding of a personal faith in Christ is possible. The other churches in this group, like the previous groups, baptise infants (although some individual ministers also recognise believer's

baptisms). In emergencies, the requirements are similar to the other churches who baptise newly-born babies whose lives are threatened. There is less emphasis upon the need for the baptism of a dying child. The parent's desires and beliefs should be honoured.

Infant dedication or presentation

Those who do not baptise infants have an infant dedication or presentation service. Where the parents request such a service at the bedside in an emergency, the appropriate chaplain or minister should be called. The short service includes Bible readings and prayer appropriate for the occasion.

Holy communion

these churches regularly celebrate services of holy communion. The patient may request communion and the chaplain or minister available is able to accede to the request.

Anointing of the sick

This is practised with varying degrees of acceptance and regularity. There is a growing practice of a healing ministry through anointing. It is almost invariably performed at the request of the patient. The chaplain or minister, with elders or deacons present, conducts the anointing.

The Order of St. Luke, which has supporters from most denominations including Catholic, established and free churches, holds a balanced stance on anointing and healing of the sick. Representatives may be called in by relatives for anointing and prayers of healing. The pentecostal and neo-charismatic churches strongly hold to a position of faith healing. Caution should be exercised with people who see illness as denomic and stress the need for "deliverance" through exorcism.

Last anointing

There are no last rites. The chaplain or minister prefers to be called to be with the patients and relatives before death takes place. The chaplain or minister considers it a privileged ministry at the bedside of the one dying, to be with the relatives, offering prayer, comfort and support.

(e) Others

Church of the Latter-Day Saints (Mormons): if the patient requires a sacrament, the State president or church leader will provide the sacrament each Sunday upon notification.

Jehovah's Witnesses do not celebrate sacraments such as baptism, anointing, holy communion. On each eve of Jewish Passover they celebrate the death of Christ in a eucharistic type of service. This is their only sacramental form of service.

II DIET AND FASTING

(a) Catholics

Usually Catholics are required to fast as preparation for Holy Communion; as a penance; during the season of Lent; or as any other worthy spiritual exercise or form of devotion.

These are not always observed by Catholics these days.

Some may make special efforts during Lent,

which are looked upon as a self-denial. They may abstain from eating meat on the first day of Lent and all the Fridays of Lent. Patients may inform hospital staff of any such special devotions. However, most would not insist upon following these in hospital.

Where medical and therapeutic reasons suggest otherwise, the Catholic is *not* obliged to conform to the usual church regulations in regard to these matters of fast and abstinence. (In fact, the patient may be conscience-bound not to follow the regulations in order to aid the healing process.)

(b) Orthodox

A seriously ill patient may be excused from following dietary obligations during Lent. During this period an Orthodox person is expected to abstain from meat and all animal produce, e.g. milk, cheese, butter, eggs.

(c), (d) Established & Non-conformist churches

Generally there are no obligatory dieting restrictions. However, some may personally practice abstinence and fasting. Seventh-Day Adventists ban the use of tobacco and alcohol; the use of tea and coffee is discouraged. For them a modified vegetarian diet, which includes dairy products such as milk, butter, cheese and eggs, is recommended. The eating of flesh is discouraged and the consumption of scripturally-forbidden food is not permitted. The practice of vegetarianism is widely varied and is regarded as a health matter rather than religious regulation. The dietary desires of an Adventist should be something that staff ascertain on admission.

(e) Others

The Church of Latter-Day Saints (Mormons) follow a dietary code that carries the weight of a commandment. Alcohol, tea, coffee, tobacco and cola drinks are to be avoided; although they are not vegetarians, they are encouraged to eat meat sparingly.

III CARE OF THE ILL AND DYING

All Christian denominations desire the offer of pastoral and spiritual care to their hospitalised parishioners. The local minister or priest will endeavour to make contact with known church members or may use lay pastoral care people to follow the patient's stay in hospital. It is during the period prior to death that the sacramental ministries of baptism, reconciliation (confession) and anointing should be administered. Where the sacrament of anointing is practised, this may be administered several times.

Sacramental ministry, as indicated earlier, has highest priority in the Catholic and Orthodox churches. Established churches also offer their members holy communion during their hospital stay. The other churches and the Mormons offer the lord's supper (communion) upon request.

In the Western world, hospital procedures are based generally on Christian practice. Generally there are no special procedural requirements necessary following death. Most ministers or priests would prefer to be called to see the patient and meet the family prior to the death so that more effective care of the family after death may be offered.

All churches would emphasise the dignity of the human body alive or dead. Each body should be handled with the greatest care respecting this dignity. Normal hospital procedures for handling the body after death are acceptable to all Christian churches.

IV AUTOPSIES, TRANSFUSIONS, TRANSPLANTS

Considering always the emphasis upon the dignity of the body, there are no religious objections to the conducting of an autopsy, administering blood transfusions or the donation or receipt of organs for transplantation.

An important exception are the Jehovah's Witnesses, however, who are opposed to blood transfusions. A Witness receiving a transfusion will be excommunicated.

Where a Catholic patient has any doubt or question of conscience in any of these matters it ought to be discussed with a Catholic priest. The priest has the necessary competence to advise, inform or guide the person who is faced with such difficulties.

As a basic principle, with a few exceptions, Christian churches leave decisions on these matters to the individual conscience of the professional and the patient.

V ABORTION AND FAMILY PLANNING

Here we find the churches at variance in their belief and practice. Most believe that human life begins at conception and that interference with the normal development raises moral, ethical and legal issues of considerable weight and that any decision on abortion should not be made without due consideration of these.

(a) Catholic Group

In general the Catholic church *rejects* the following on moral grounds: Abortion—no matter how early it is; aborti-facient procedures, drugs etc.; the contraceptive pill, creams, devices (I.U.D.); tubal ligation; vasectomy or any other form or method of sterilisation.

The church recognises the so-called Natural family planning method, which is built upon the ovulation cycle. ("With this method it is possible for a couple to avoid the 'contraceptive' mentality... Rather it encourages a spirit of responsible parenthood which a couple can use right from the first day of their marriage together". Thus responsible parenthood was advanced and advocated by Pope Paul VI in his Encyclical *Humanae Vitae* (1968).)

Where medical circumstances raise the question of need for the termination of a pregnancy, a Catholic couple may seek a consultation with a Catholic priest to enable a decision in good faith and with a peaceful conscience.

(b) Orthodox Group

The Syrian Orthodox church considers abortion in all its forms to be wrong—"simply murder". A pregnant woman should not consent to an operation which threatens the life of a child without consulting the priest.

The Greek Orthodox position is similar in prohibiting any medical procedure which would terminate the life of the foetus or embryo. However, in case of haemorrhage, procedures designed to stop the bleeding as distinct from procedures for expelling the living attached foetus are permissible, even if foetal death eventuates.

(c), (d), (e) Established, Non-conformist and other groups

These churches stand for the sacredness of human life. The moral and ethical dilemmas in this area are understood. "Abortion on demand" would not be officially condoned. A termination of pregnancy is mostly acceptable if, for medical reasons, the mother's life is in danger. As a form of birth control it is unacceptable. The mother or couple's right to make a judgement with a clear conscience is often the accepted procedure after a sincere consideration of the ethical issues involved in the case.

The advance of modern medical knowledge and technology raises the ethical problems in such matters as surrogate motherhood, artificial insemination by a donor and in-vitro fertilisation. These have left the churches in a position where they cannot offer definitive answers in theology.

Each circumstance must be considered in its uniqueness and left to the individual conscience. These churches generally have no problems with the use of contraceptives and other procedures in birth control and family planning.

VI MODESTY

All denominations of the Christian church recognise the sacredness and dignity of the human body and accept the need for the treatment of that body with modesty. This sense of modesty will vary from individual to individual and from generation to generation. Some female patients might prefer to be cared for by a female doctor and nurse, but these days health care professionals are able to meet the needs of all patients without embarrassment. Where agitation on the grounds of modesty is shown or expressed, staff should be allocated accordingly, if possible, showing due respect.

3. Islam

The word "Allah" is the Arabic word for God. Muslims, Christians and Jews worship the one God. The roots of the three religions go back to the time before Abraham, who is the common link.

"Islam" means "submission" or "the act of submitting oneself"; "Muslim", from the same root, carries the meaning "one who submits". Therefore a Muslim is one who submits to Allah.

A follower of Islam is not a Mohammadan, but a Muslim. The use of the former term or its equivalent is likely to cause offence.

Mohammad (peace be upon him), the founder of Islam, was born 570 AD at Mecca. At age 40 he went into a desert cave to meditate. In the last days of the month of Ramadan he received a vision. This and later revelations became the basis of the Qu'ran, or Koran. Non-acceptance of his teaching caused his flight to Medina in 622 AD. Later that year 300 of his followers defeated an army of 1000 men. Thus *jihad*, or holy war, began. In 630 AD with 10 000 armed men he captured Mecca. Thus the Islamic faith was established. He died in Medina in 632 AD and is believed to be the final prophet.

Mohammed (peace be upon him) prescribed a special way of life and rules known as the Five Pillars of Islam:

- *Confession of Faith* daily in front of witnesses: "There is no God but Allah and Mohammad is his prophet".
- *Prayer* five times a day facing Mecca and with prescribed washing, ritual and gestures.
- *Fasting* during the month of Ramadan: for 28 days, no healthy Muslim may eat, drink or smoke between dawn and sunset.
- *Almsgiving*, a sign of Islamic brotherhood.
- *Pilgrimage to Mecca*, known as the *haj*.

The absolute singularity of Allah (monotheism) is the basis of the Muslim's concept of God. He is the creator, controller and governor of the universe. A believer's life and property belong to God. The fear of life, personal safety, or pain demonstrates a lack of belief and submission to Allah. Everything that happens in a person's life has been determined by Allah within the first forty days of conception. Complaint against the vagaries of life is considered as criticism of Allah's will for the individual. (It is not uncommon for a Muslim to interrupt a sentence to say in Arabic "Praise be to Allah" or "Thanks be to Allah" (*hum'dullah*) every time there is a twinge of pain. This is to be seen as a gracious acceptance of the pain planned by Allah).

As Allah is the controller of human lives, he is also the provider of all things necessary to fulfil his will in a person's life. Muslims therefore often do not show fear and doubt about their hospitalisation.

Muslims are appalled at the permissive Western "Christian" society. They are continually warning their people not to lower their own moral standards in family matters, sexual looseness, alcohol consumption, dress, gambling, etc. Some Muslims who have become more integrated into Western society have moderated their living style, which is causing concern to Muslim leaders. These fears and concerns may be carried into the hospital. Such tensions are to be noted and assurances of respect for Islamic beliefs and practices indicated by staff.

DIET AND FASTING

The eating of pork, bacon, ham, or any other by-product of pork is strictly forbidden, nor should these items come into contact with any other food which is to be eaten by Muslims. Alcohol is totally forbidden, even its use in small quantities in preparing meals, puddings or cakes.

Muslims are allowed to eat beef, mutton and poultry provided the meat is halal (killed and prepared by a Muslim according to Islamic law). There are no restrictions on fish, vegetables, dairy products and fruit.

Some Muslims may refuse to eat hospital food and may insist on having food brought into them. The older generation is usually very conservative. In co-operation with hospital staff, patients or their relatives may be consulted to ascertain any dietary preferences, as hospital food may prove unappetising for Muslims, who often prefer spicy foods.

Ramadan is usually a month of fasting. Fasting is not required of the sick, the traveller, and nursing mothers. The two big Muslim festivals are the Eed-ul-Fitr, which ends Ramadan, and Eed-ul-Azha which commences the *haj* (pilgrimage to Mecca). This Eed also commemorates Abraham's willingness to offer his son as a sacrifice. (The Muslim tradition identifies the son of Ishmael, Hagar's son, and not Isaac, Sarah's son.) The family may request that the patient be given leave to go home for these two days. Like Christmas cards, Eed cards are sent. Wishing the patient a happy Eed by the staff is appreciated as an expression of goodwill to Muslim patients.

Examinations, tests and surgery should be avoided, if possible, on an Eed day.

PASTORAL AND SPIRITUAL CARE

In Islam it is mandatory for an imam or spiritual leader to visit the sick in hospital if called. If there is a request for an imam, mulvi or sheikh, the request must be followed through. In practice many imams are in secular employment and carry out their duties as teachers at the Friday mosque prayers. As their time is limited, they may not be able to visit the patient in hospital. The reciting of special portions of the Koran under certain conditions is necessary. These may be recited and prayers offered by relatives or friends. Any prayers offered by an imam are in Koranic form. They do not name the patient as this would be deemed a criticism of Allah's will for the patient.

Prayers form a Christian minister or official pastoral care person may be acceptable, as Jesus is the only healing prophet in the Koran.

AUTOPSIES, TRANSPLANTS TRANSUFUSIONS

Routine or non-essential autopsies are not permitted. Where it is necessary for the issue of a death certificate or for coronial purposes an autopsy is accepted. As the body is to be resurrected on the last day, it should be buried intact. Thus organ donations are not made generally. However, organ transplants may be received where medical need dictates. Blood transfusions are acceptable for Muslim patients.

RITUALS

Birth
No religious sacrament or ritual is required except that a member of the child's family recite a prayer in the baby's ear as soon as convenient after the birth.

Arrangements should be made for the circumcision of a male child as soon as possible after the birth. Comments by hospital staff criticising the practice is considered distasteful and unprofessional.

Ritual ablutions and washing
Muslims have strict rules for ritual washing and hygiene practice.

Mosques provide adequate water for purification before prayers. Cleanliness for them is important. Preparation for worship, for instance, includes the washing three times of face, ears, forehead, feet to ankles, hands, arms to elbows, the sniffing of water up the nose and washing out the mouth. Wet hands are rubbed through the hair to remove dust. A devout Muslim may wish to do this five times a day, although exemption because of illness is possible.

In personal cleanliness showering is preferable to a bath. Toilets should be provided with a jug which can be filled with water as Muslims need to wash their private parts after urination or defecation. It is not possible to pray without this washing.

ABORTION AND FAMILY PLANNING

Birth control would generally be considered an endeavour to circumvent Allah's will for life. Pressure to practice birth control should not be asserted, rather it should be explained. According to the degree of westernisation, devotion, education or economic circumstances, the need for birth control will be considered.

Abortion is forbidden unless the mother's physical and mental health are in danger.

CARE OF THE ILL AND DYING

A dying Muslim may desire to sit or lie facing Mecca: that is, north-west in Australia to New Zealand; south-west in the United Kingdom and Europe; west to south-west in North America. The movement of the bed to such a position is deeply appreciated. Relatives may recite portions of the Koran around

the bed. If there are no relatives, then any Muslim
may offer such help and comfort.

As the patient is dying, a pillow should be put
under the head to elevate it above the rest of the
body. The Muslim call to prayer, the "Kalima",
should be recited by friends. Sura (chapter) 36 of
the Koran is also appropriate: it ends "all glory to
Him who controls all things! Unto Him you shall all
return".

Even though there is an acceptance of and an
acknowledged submission to Allah's plan for their
life and his timing of their death, many Muslims are
fearful when dying. May be it is a fear of their state in
the future life. On which rung of the ladder of seven
hells and seven heavens will they find themselves?
Death is a taboo subject for Muslims.

Grief counselling is not well accepted. It may
even be considered an intrusion of privacy. A dying
patient may show passivity, which may be for one of
three reasons: a resigned acceptance of their fate;
disguised fear, since fear would indicate lack of
trust in Allah's judgement and mercy; or guilt over
inadequate submission prior to illness. They pas-
sively accept the perceived punishment for their
sins of commission and omission.

Expressions of grief vary according to the age and
sex of the dying patient. Slapping, scratching and
punching the body as expressions of grief are
encountered and condoned. They are, however,
contrary to Muslim belief. To mar the body which
Allah made is an affront to Allah.

Regarding euthanasia, Muslims would consider
the stopping of medical procedures as a contraven-
tion of Allah's will for the patient's life. The timing of
death is in Allah's hands.

Handling of the deceased body

Only Muslims if possible should handle the body in hospital—a male for a male, a female for a female. If a Muslim is not available, then non-Muslims should use disposable gloves so as not to touch the body.

The eyes should be closed; the lower jaw should be bandaged to the head to stop a gaping mouth. The body is then straightened. The limbs and joints are first flexed several times before being placed in final position. The body should not be washed, hair or nails cut; the body should be covered, the head turned right, to face Mecca when buried.

The body is removed by a funeral director authorised by the Islamic community, who will wash and prepare the body for burial according to Muslim procedures.

If there is any doubt, the local Muslim community should be consulted.

MODESTY

Nakedness is anathema to a Muslim and hospitalisation does not lessen the sensitivity. Women usually are fully covered from head to foot, even in bed, so that their body form may not be seen. The requirement to don only a hospital gown for surgery or other reasons is likely to be met with opposition.

Some Muslim women may refuse an internal examination prior to birth.

Men always remain covered from waist to knee. Any less clothing even in front of other men is offensive.

Medical examinations of patients in front of a number of doctors and students of both sexes is objectionable.

This attitude can, of course, create problems for hospital staff. Male Muslims should be examined by men. Similarly only female nurses and doctors should examine Muslim women. More conservative Muslim males may have a second objection to females being in charge of their medical or nursing care. They may object to the concept of a woman having a position over them about which they can do little.

Again, older devout males may wish to keep their head covered at all times. Staff should respect this desire, not making any fuss or reference to it.

A SIGNIFICANT CULTURAL DIFFERENCE

Many Muslim cultural groups have strict procedures concerning the discussion of medical information with family and patient. Second-degree male relatives of the patient, e.g. uncles and cousins, should be informed of any diagnosis, procedure and prognosis. They in turn consider the wisdom or otherwise of telling the patient and immediate family. Our Western society and medical practice find this objectionable as it runs counter to the civil rights of the patient. Some Muslims, however, prefer it to be this way. Patients then do not have to contemplate the future life at that stage and this enables them to proceed through the illness without the resigned acceptance already mentioned, disguised fear or guilt. Doctors and nursing staff would be wise to ascertain the family's desires in information sharing. Such acknowledgement is likely to bring far

greater cooperation and support of the medical
team by the relatives. It would be wise to lay some
ground rules by identifying the persons to be told
and limiting their number to two or three.

4. Judaism

Judaism is the first of the great monotheistic religions of the world. About 2000 BC, Abraham, who was of Sumerian background, came out from Mesopotamia to settle in the Palestine area of the Levant. Between 1700 and 1200 BC, the descendants of his grandson, Israel, were enslaved in Egypt. Moses miraculously led the children of Israel, escaping the slavery, into 40 years of wilderness wanderings before settling down, according to the promise of God, in Palestine. During these years by divine revelation Moses received the Jewish law, including the Ten Commandments, which has become the basis of the religion. Numerous other laws or traditions have been amassed as interpretations and applications of those laws. The basic law is the Torah, or the Pentateuch, which is found in the first five books of the Old Testament; a portion is read every Sabbath.

do not recognise Jesus Christ as the Messiah. There are orthodox, liberal and new conservative Jews who observe the law with varying degrees of literalism. The rabbi or minister called to a patient should be from the same school as the family.

Sabbath is from sunset on Friday evening to sunset Saturday evening or from the first sighting of three stars. Orthodox Jews strictly observe it as a day of rest. Attendance at synagogue, saying of prayers, the lighting of candles are all part of Sabbath worship. There are certain limitations as to what may or may not be done on the Sabbath, depending upon the degree of orthodoxy or the rabbinical school followed.

The Jews have had a history of dispersion across the known world from 722 BC onwards. In many countries they have been forced to live in ghettos and maintained strict solidarity. In others, although they retained their distinctiveness, there has been a greater integration and a weakening of their conservatism. The strict orthodox Jews still wear eighteenth-century dress and have uncut hair. In places like Jerusalem they are readily identified. As a result of the dispersion many have adopted the food habits, dress and codes of conduct of the adopted lands. This makes it all the more important for hospital staff to ascertain the special religious requirements, if any, that need to be observed during their hospitalisation.

RITUAL

As already noted, the Sabbath should be observed as a day of rest. Some strict orthodox Jews will prefer not to write or switch on or off electric appliances on the Sabbath. If bed lights, radio or television are turned on for them it is appreciated. The majority of Jews would accept normal hospital routine.

Pastoral and spiritual care

Visiting the sick is a supreme commandment for followers of the Jewish faith. It is incumbent not only on family members, but on all Jews, especially those who are friends or neighbours of the sick. It should be undertaken in a genuine spirit of warm and practical concern for the needs of patients, giving them reassurance and comfort in the hours of pain and weakness. The best help often is prayer— for the sick and with the sick.

Ministers gratefully appreciate the co-operation of hospital staff and Jewish colleagues in the ministry in assisting them by notifications, particularly of emergencies, and in other practical ways.

DIET

Dietary requirements of Jewish hospital patients will depend on the degree of observance customary in their homes. Those patients who uphold the special dietary laws (Kashrut) will do so also in hospital. Very briefly, these laws refer to the provision of kosher food—special slaughtering and preparation of meat, separation of milk and meat foods, forbidden food, etc. In the period of Passover, avoidance of all leaven and the provision of unleavened bread (matzah) is essential.

To obviate any difficulties for such observing in hospitals, the following points are important:

- In co-operation with hospital staff, and with medical approval, the family concerned may be allowed to bring kosher food into hospital;
- Milk and meat are usually not eaten at the same meal. Up to six hours may be required between eating meat and dairy produce;
- Some patients may be satisfied with the provision of vegetarian food, including dairy foods;
- A kosher meals service - if and when available - provide certain prepackaged meals by private arrangement (contact a rabbi or synagogue for information);
- In cases of danger to life, dietary laws are temporarily suspended;
- The assistance of a Jewish minister is particularly desirable and should be sought by dietitians at hospitals where patients have food problems.

CARE OF THE ILL AND DYING

A basic tenet of Judaism emphasises that nothing must be allowed to stand in the way of preserving or prolonging life. Sabbath observance may be waived if necessary to assist a person whose life is in danger.

God himself is the supreme physician, "Who healeth the broken-hearted and bindeth up their wounds" (*Psalm* 147:3). Nevertheless, it is readily conceded that the divine healer does his work through mortals, and high respect is shown to members of the medical profession, following Ben Sira's famous utterance: "Honour a physician according to thy need of him, with the honours due unto him; for verily the Lord hath created him" (*Ecclesiasticus* 38:1-2).

Faith-healing, as it is understood in a specific sense by some Christians is foreign, and unknown within, Judaism.

It is the doctor's duty to prolong life, so euthanasia is contrary to Jewish teachings. *No direct action to hasten death is permitted.* A patient on life support systems should remain on them until death. All active treatment should be maintained.

The Jewish religion does not recognise the concept of sacrament in the sense in which it is used by Christians. A person approaching death is encouraged to confess his or her sins before God (*Viddui* or confession) and to evoke God's forgiveness. No confessor is needed, in the Jewish view, since only God can absolve sin. The shortest formula is: "May my death atone for my transgressions", but this and other more elaborate wordings are best prompted and recited with the dying by a minister in attendance.

It is a basic tenet of Judaism that a dying person should not be left alone. When the end approaches, the last paragraph of the confession should be recited, especially "Hear O Israel, the Lord our God, the Lord is One".

The reading of Psalm 23 and the saying of the prayer (the *shema*) may be desired.

If at all possible, a minister of the Jewish faith (hospital chaplain or local rabbi or reverend) should be called in time to attend to the needs of the dying patient.

Handling the deceased body

Death is presumed to occur when breathing appears to have stopped. When it is finally established, the eyes and mouth are gently closed (preferably by a near relative).

When life has departed, the arms and hands are extended at the side of the body. The lower jaw is bound up. The body is then placed on the floor with the feet towards the door and is covered with a sheet, while a lighted candle is placed close to the head.

The body must not be moved on the Sabbath (from Friday evening sunset to Saturday evening sunset, plus 30 minutes approximately). If death occurs in a hospital or nursing home, and no fellow Jews are available to carry out these services, they may be carried out by hospital staff.

There is in most Jewish communities a special association, called Chevra Kadisha (Holy Brotherhood), which concerns itself with the burial of the dead. It is essential that this association which functions as the Jewish burial society be notified immediately when a death occurs.

The Chevra will take charge of all arrangements from the moment of notification. It will, in particular, remove the dead and will see to all other rites: ritual purification, including washing, shrouds, provision of the coffin, and all further funeral arrangements.

It will not operate on Sabbaths and festivals, but special provisions apply once the Association is contacted.

Orthodox Jews are always buried in special Jewish burial grounds. Some liberal Jews may choose cremation.

AUTOPSIES, TRANSFUSIONS, TRANSPLANTS

It is forbidden in Jewish law to carry out an *autopsy* to ascertain the cause of death unless it is ordered by civil authorities. *Dissection*, including dissection for organs for donation, is regarded as dishonouring the human body. Some Jewish authorities, however, do not object to organ transplants provided that no organ is removed until death has been established.

The Chief Rabbinate of the State of Israel sanctions a post-mortem examination when it is legally required, when in the opinion of three doctors the cause of death cannot otherwise be ascertained, when it might help or save the lives of others suffering from similar maladies* or in case of certain hereditary diseases.

This ruling would be broadly applicable in all Jewish communities.

Blood transfusions, if required and authorised by medical staff in the interests of the patient's welfare and life prolongation, are permitted. The patient's and family's preferences in these matters must be ascertained.

Eye transplants are permitted by some authorities under certain safeguards on the grounds that they will help to restore sight to the living. An express request concerning this may be obeyed.

*The Chief Rabbinate of Israel does not object to the use of bodies for anatomical dissection as required for medical studies, provided earlier voluntary consent has been given by the person concerned, and provided the dissected parts are carefully preserved for later burial.

ABORTION AND FAMILY PLANNING

Contraception

Mechanical methods of contraception are not favoured. Oral methods of birth control are acceptable. Sperm for IVF programmes must be from the husband. Orthodox Jews are more strict in their attitudes, therefore all forms of sterilisation are forbidden. Reformed Jews are more accepting.

Abortion is a complex problem in the Jewish Law with no clear-cut answer. The following points are essential:

- Up to the moment of the first signs of labour, the foetus is an organic part of the mother. The artificial termination of pregnancy—whilst not an act of murder—is strongly condemned on moral grounds, unless it can be justified for medical reasons (serious deformity, imbecility and similar causes);
- The foetus must be destroyed if this is the only way in which the mother's life can be saved;
- Abortion for economic reasons, or where the child is unwanted, is not permitted.

Circumcision

On the birth of a male child, the parents' Rabbi should be notified to arrange the ritual circumcision. Any doubt about the child's health will delay the circumcision. The rite is conducted by a trained and medically certified religious person, often the local Rabbi. Should the mother and child still be in hospital, a private room should be made available. A quorum (usually 10) Jewish males should be present.

MODESTY

An orthodox Jewess will dress circumspectly and would prefer to have her body and limbs covered. She may refuse to permit herself to be uncovered for examination for teaching purposes. A woman may wear a wig or scarf so that others will not see her hair.

Male staff may attend female patients within the rules and framework of routine hospital arrangements which safeguard accepted standards of decency and modesty. While this is broadly the accepted position, it is possible that some Jewish patients may still object for religious reasons, and in such rare cases hospital staff will undoubtedly show understanding and co-operation.

5. Hinduism

Hinduism is probably the oldest of the recognised living religions. It is difficult to date its origins, but to suggest that it is more than 4000 years since establishment would not be an over-estimation.

Hinduism embraces a galaxy of gods and goddesses. Ancient scriptures such as the Vedas, the Upanishads, the Brahmanas, the Bhagavad Gita and other epics, such as the Mahabharata and the Ramayana, contain rich stories of these deities.

Basically Hindus believe in an ultimate great spirit, Brahman or Atma. He may be worshipped in many forms. Then comes the trimurti consisting of Brahma, the creator; Vishnu, the preserver and Shib or Shiva, the destroyer and regenerator of life. After these comes a myriad of avatars and other deities.

Each major deity represents certain aspects of human living such as the elephant-headed Ganash, the god of wealth. At the back of the till storekeepers often keep a shrine to Ganesh, with incense burning, Saraswati is the goddess of learning and is worshipped at the commencement of the school year in most public schools and even homes where there are school age children.

Certain areas of India place a greater emphasis upon a particular god or goddess. For instance the goddess durga, the victor over evil, is the main deity worshipped in eastern India, particularly Bengal.

Originally the Hindu caste system was an ideal way of ensuring a living and employment for all. The castes were the first form of trade union or work guilds. In India it is now illegal although some customs die hard.

The doctrine of karma (the moral law of cause and effect) influences many a Hindu's attitude to life. Hindus see life events as being due to his karma. Many interpret this as fatalism. Karma is the working out in this present life of something that happened in a past life. Strongly believing in reincarnation, they hold that present status and behaviour have a bearing on existence in the next reincarnated life.

Hinduism may be looked upon as a philosophy which covers the whole of life, including health. Ayurvedic medicine, practised for millennia, is still practised today. A Hindu may show some reticence to follow protocol in hospital in case it counters ayurvedic practice, which covers a regimen of regular diet, sleep, defaecation, hygiene, clothing, exercise and sexual practice.

Practitioners of ayurvedic medicine are recognised as being experts, who are honest and trustworthy. Such trust and confidence may be transferred from the ayurvedic doctor to the doctor of Western medicine.

Because of the belief in reincarnation, orthodox Hindus are vegetarians. In reincarnation, the spirit of a newly-deceased person may enter a dog, cow, chicken, even an egg. However westernisation sometimes weakens these beliefs and practices.

The Hindu's ultimate hope is to live such a good life in one of her or his many incarnations that she or he will eventually be absorbed into Brahman (Atma). By living a pure ethical life, loving and caring for fellow human beings and other creatures, "humans can realise God".

Hindu worship consists of a plethora of rituals which are focused in the family shrine, the local temple and a pilgrimage site. The household shrine is set up within the home or in the courtyard or it may be the *tulsi* (basil) bush growing in the court-yard, around which the instruments for worship are arranged. At dusk each evening the women usually perform *puja* around the shrine, their distinctive wail resounding around the village accompanied by the ringing of bells and the waving of incense. Prayers are offered for the personal needs of the family. The local temple is visited by some on a regular basis and on particular festival days for the temple deity when the whole community joins in. Places of special pilgrimage are found from Arma-nath in the Kashmir Himalayas to Karmakhya in Assam to Varanasi by the Ganges.

The times of *puja*, or worship, are important as worshippers believe they are encountering the for-ces that influence the physical and material world—the worshipper's world. Such worship practices are not possible in the hospital ward. The family, partic-ularly the women, will visit their own temple or conduct *puja* around the family altar at home.

NAMES

Hindu patients are likely to have three or four names, according to their background. In the north it is usual to have a given or personal (not Christian) name followed by a second one, possibly the father's given name or the name of a deity or a title, e.g. Bipendra (father's name), Chandra (moon), Krishna (god) or Kumar (Prince). The third name is the family name, which usually indicates the caste, e.g. Chakraborty (brahman or priestly caste), Agawalla (merchant caste). In south India four names may be used: great-grandfather, grandfather, father and given name. The last name should always be used for medical records.

DIET AND FASTING

For most Hindus diet is important. Most will not eat beef; vegetarian Hindus eat no white or red meats, no eggs, and nothing that is produced from animals. Some, however, may eat cottage cheese, yoghurt, even eggs and drink milk. Tomato or similar sandwiches are safe to offer a Hindu patient. There are certain other eating taboos with certain types of illnesses.

Always enquire carefully of a Hindu's dietary needs.

Fasting is not considered obligatory in hospital during festival periods. There are those few who may insist on fasting, but even in this case tea, hot milk, salt-free salads and fruits are permitted. At the end of the festival relatives may bring in food and sweetmeats that have been offerings for the *puja*.

RITUALS

Birth

Birth practices vary. In the higher caste families the mother is forced to rest for forty days after the birth.

For the pious Hindu three ceremonies take place before birth:

- to promote conception
- to procure a male child
- to ensure the safety of the child in the womb.

In the home birth, a ceremony involving mantras (prayer) said in the baby's ear, putting a mixture of honey and ghee (clarified butter) on the baby's tongue, and naming her or him is followed. The name is kept secret until later.

This birth scenario is not possible in a hospital. However, the mantra and name may be whispered in the baby's ear as soon as possible after birth by the mother or father. It requires only one or two minutes.

Where hospital procedures insist on moving the baby into a nursery it may require considerable persuasion to pacify the separated mother.

Ritual ablutions and washing

Physical cleansing is associated with spiritual cleansing; hence its importance to the Hindu. As with most people of Asian origin, there will be the need for water for washing after use of the toilet. A container of water should be available in the toilet and when a bedpan is used. Hindus, like Muslims, prefers showers or running water to baths.

AUTOPSIES, TRANSFUSIONS, TRANSPLANTS

There are no religious objections to such procedures. Autopsies generally are acceptable although Hindus are happier if they can be avoided. Only normal consent procedures for organ donation or transplants need to be followed.

However, some may object strongly to post-mortems and organ donations, desiring the body to remain intact.

ABORTION AND FAMILY PLANNING

Hinduism places no restriction on the use of contraception. The importance of a male child to a family may put pressure upon the woman to continue with additional pregnancies until a son is born. If there are medical or financial reasons for the limitation of the size of the family, then the husband should be involved in any such information-sharing and decision-making.

CARE OF THE ILL AND DYING

In an area with a strong Hindi community, a Hindu priest is able to help in matters of worship (*puja*). Accepting death philosophically is a trait of Hinduism; the priest, if available, fulfills the role of facilitating such acceptance. A devout Hindu may desire to read or hear the Hindu scriptures, particularly the Bhagavad Gita.

Other rituals that may be performed are: the tying of a thread around the neck or wrist of the dying patient, the sprinkling of Ganges water over the patient, the placing of a leaf from the sacred basil (tulsi) bush on the tongue, or the bringing of money for the patient to touch before it is offered as alms to the needy.

Some patients may want to lie on the floor to be closer to the earth with incense burning around them. Patience is required in handling them. Others may want to die at home. Every reasonable consideration should be given to such a request.

Handling of the decreased body

Following death, the family should be consulted before the body is handled as the family may wish to wash and dress the deceased. Where such consultation is not possible, disposable gloves should be used to close the eyes and straighten the limbs and remove jewellery.

*Sacred threads and other religious objects should not be removed. The body—unwashed, as this is part of the family funeral rites—should be wrapped in a plain sheet or shroud. It will be cremated.

Hindu practice varies widely. The above is only a general outline of what may be expected. Always ask the patient or eldest son or other senior male relatives what the patient's wishes are or would be.

*The sacred thread is presented to a son of the brahman (priestly) caste. It is a white thread tied around the waist and up over the shoulder. The patient should be cremated wearing the sacred thread.

MODESTY

Hindu women may indicate a preference to be treated or examined by a female doctor.

Efforts should be made to avoid the embarrassment to a patient being sent for tests in a short hospital gown.

6. Sikhism

In Hinduism, the power of ritual, the effectiveness of mantras, the sacrificial system unifies the people under the power of the priests. Mahavira, the founder of Jainism, and Siddarth Gautama, founder of Buddhism, argued that the priestly dominance did not permit the ordinary worshippers to understand truth and receive enlightenment or liberation. Hence they separated from Hinduism a few centuries before the Christian era.

Two thousand years later Guru Nanak (1469-1539) saw the caste system as dangerous, other elements as too complicated and also perceived that ritual dominated. Influenced by Islam (and perhaps Christianity), he recognised the confusion created by a multiplicity of gods. His reform renounced the priesthood, the caste system and established monotheism. He also gave women a new status. Equality of all people became a focal point. Sikhism is more than a reform of Hinduism; Nanak and his nine successors developed an independent religion. They retained the Hindu concept of reincarnation until true understanding and unity with the divine is accomplished.

The writings of the ten prophets or gurus form the Sikh scriptures known as Guru Grant Sahab, or Ad Granth. Sikhs use this as their teacher as there is no priesthood. The Sikh Gurdwara (temple) is managed by the community, who oversee all religious and social services.

Guru Gobind Singh (1666-1780) was the last of the gurus. It was he who developed the militaristic character of the Sikhs. He also built upon Nanak's emphasis upon the equality of the sexes, which differed greatly from Hinduism and Islam.

Gobind Singh takes the credit for establishing the wearing of the five K symbols by every initiated Sikh male or female. There should be an awareness of these symbols when nursing or treating a Sikh, to avoid embarrassment or misunderstanding. They are:

Kesh—uncut hair. Usually it is left long and tied into a bun. The men cover it with a turban; elderly pious Sikh women may wear black turbans.

Kangha—a comb. A small semi-circular comb to keep the bun in place. Even if for some medical or surgical reason it cannot be kept in the bun it should always remain close to the patient's body.

Kara—a steel bangle. Originally used to protect the wrist from cuts from the bow string, it now symbolises the unity of God. During surgery it should not be removed but covered, as with a wedding ring. Where the arm on which it is worn is involved in the procedure, the bangle can be put on the other wrist, worn pinned to the pyjamas or put under the pillow.

Kirpan—a short dagger. It symbolises the readiness of the Sikh to fight against injustice and to protect the oppressed. Some Sikhs still carry a real dagger. More commonly worn as a brooch or pendant, *Kirpan* may also be engraved on the *Kangha*. Sikhs who wear the Kirpan will wear it all the time in bed, under the shower and in hospital. To remove it will cause great distress to the patient. If in exceptional circumstances it cannot be worn against the body, it must be kept in sight. The reasons must be carefully *explained to the patient and relatives and be understood* by them.

Kaccha—white underpants or shorts. Originally these were knee-length for ease of movement in battle. They also symbolise modesty and sexual morality. At child birth a woman may insist on having one leg in a *Kaccha*. In changing *Kacchas* one leg must remain in the old or soiled *Kaccha* until the other leg is in the clean one. This should be observed when giving a bed bath or a bedpan.

NAMES

The Sikhs usually have three names. There is the given name first, e.g. Mahinda for a male or Amrit for a female. Then comes a title, Singh for all men and Kaur for all women. A family name such as Gill or Bhuller then follows.

Thus a man's name may be Mahinda Singh Gill.

He will often register as Mahinda Gill Singh; similarly a woman as Amrit Bhuller Kaur. To keep medical records from confusion, it is wiser to register patients under the family name as Gill, M. S. or Bhuller A. K. A husband is usually known as Mr Singh and his wife as Mrs Kaur; never Mrs Singh.

RITUAL

For devout Sikhs prayer is important. Normally a Sikh will rise early, bathe and say prayers before breakfast. In hospital, privacy is essential when saying prayers. The following should be made available if possible, even for a dying patient:

- the opportunity for an early shower or
- a quick bed sponge before prayers at breakfast
- the pulling of curtains to ensure privacy whilst praying

DIET AND FASTING

There is a wide range of practices. Most of the official Sikh stances relating to food and drink are now observed, but with varying degrees of strictness.

Some common restrictions ban:
- alcohol
- halal meat
- eggs, for many women who are vegetarian
- beef or pork
- tobacco smoking.

Since not all Sikhs observe the above restrictions,

each Sikh patient should be asked about special requirements.

A few Sikhs may wish to fast when there is a full moon.

Ritual ablutions and washing

Running water for washing and showering with the provision of water near the toilet or with the bedpan are requirements.

Water is also required for washing the hands and mouth before eating.

Birth

Sikhs consider a woman to be at her best after childbirth and susceptible to chills and back pain at such time. She will not wish to bathe for a few days to avoid these risks. Normally a nursing mother is allowed forty days rest after the birth. Hospital routine may seem to run counter to this.

Separation of mothers from the baby into a nursery may be met with resistance. Tactful explanations will be necessary if this is hospital procedure.

Relatives and friends will want to see the baby as soon after the birth as possible and gifts of clothing are usually tried on the baby. Restraint may be necessary or gentle persuasion just to leave the gift will be needed by the staff.

ABORTION AND
FAMILY PLANNING

Abortions are acceptable only if the mother's life is at risk.

There are generally no objections to contraception and family planning.

AUTOPSIES, TRANSFUSIONS AND TRANSPLANTS

There are no religious objections to any of these.

Careful and neat suturing of the body post autopsy is required in case the family insist on washing the body prior to cremation. Careless presentation of the body is likely to cause great distress.

CARE OF THE ILL AND DYING

Sikhs may derive comfort from hearing passages of the Guru Grant Sahab when dying. If unable to read themselves a relative or any practising Sikh may do it.

Because of their belief in reincarnation, Sikhs are not fearful of death. They believe they can alter the cycle by living a good life and accumulating rewards or punishments in the next life.

Handling of the deceased body

Non-Sikhs may attend the body at death. It is essential to see that the five K's or symbols are in place and have not been mistreated. No hair should be cut or trimmed. A nurse may close the eyes and straighten out the limbs and wrap the body in a plain sheet or shroud.

Cremation takes place as soon as possible (except when there is a stillborn child, then the child may be buried). Some women will not eat until after the cremation. Women wear white as a sign of mourning. After ten days another ceremony, called the *Bhog*, is held to formally end the mourning period.

MODESTY

Most women would prefer to be examined by a female doctor, but they will not object to a male doctor's examination if a female nurse is present.

The removal of the *Kaccha* (undershorts) from either male or female may cause great embarrassment as will the removal of the turban.

7. Buddhism

A royal prince, named Siddhartha, was born in the 6th century BC in what is now the Himalayan kingdom of Nepal. This prince observed that most people experienced suffering of one kind or another and understood that people sought unsuccessfully for happiness. He left the comfort of palace and home to seek the truth that would bring true happiness.

After several years of futile search, a sudden inspiration took hold of him whilst he was sitting, meditating under a banyan tree at Gaya in North India. The truth burned within him that happiness came from changing the self from the inside. This became known as "Enlightenment". He then was given the title of Buddha, which means "the enlightened one".

His expansive teaching life followed. He taught that greed, hatred and delusion destroyed happiness. Wisdom and compassion were the secret to happiness. The ultimate state, Nirvana, which is in some ways similar to what Christians call heaven, can only be attained through an absence of desire and the achievement of perfection and no awareness of separate identity.

His eightfold path to enlightenment was: right view or understanding, right thought, right speech, right action, right livelihood, right effort, right mindfulness, right meditation. Buddhists believe in reincarnation until the absence of desire is attained. They do not believe in a god as creator and worship is the acknowledgement of an ideal.

Buddhism still embraces much of the worship, teaching and beliefs of Hinduism. The philosophy of Buddhism—of prayers, purifications, meditation, retreats and virtuous living—has attracted many people from the Western world.

DIET AND FASTING

As Buddhists are found in countries with a wide range of climates, diets vary. Many Buddhists are vegetarian because the eating of meat entails suffering to the slain animal. Some may even consider, as some Hindus do, that an animal contains a reincarnated human spirit. An awareness of the possible need for a vegetarian diet is important for those Buddhist patients.

Festivals and days of fasting vary amongst the schools of Buddhism. On the special festival days the patient may request to eat before 12 noon and not after.

RITUALS

Birth

Apart from babies born into aristocratic families, no special ceremonies are performed after the birth of a child. No special rituals are required in trauma cases.

Ritual ablutions and washing

Buddhist scriptures have no special instructions concerning washing and cleansing after attending to toilet functions. Buddhists come from various countries with varying customs, so their requirements may vary. Patients should be asked if they have special needs.

AUTOPSIES, TRANSFUSIONS, TRANSPLANTS

Buddhists have no objections to autopsies, blood transfusions or transplants. These would be considered as being of assistance in the relief of suffering or the acquiring of knowledge that may help others. The only condition is that life is not destroyed in the pursuit of these. Active euthanasia is therefore forbidden.

ABORTION

For the same reason abortion is generally condemned. Similarly, family planning may be considered as interfering with one's destiny; its practice is therefore conditional upon the couple's background.

CARING OF THE ILL AND DYING

The health care staff may be either male or female except where the patient is a monk or nun (sister). In such cases, staff of the same sex should be considered for the care of the patient.

Buddhists appreciate a visit from a monk or sister if they are available. Ask the patient for the contact person.

Buddhists often spend time in meditation before a shrine. In hospital the shrine may simply be an image of the Buddha. Staff should be aware that the patient is in meditation when a picture of the Buddha is in view of the patient. Space for such meditation should be allowed as it is a factor in physical well-being and recuperation.

There are two conflicting emphases of Buddhism which affects the patient: the relief of pain and suffering and the importance of "mindfulness", that is, being mentally alert and aware.

A patient in pain is usually offered pain relief which sedates and impairs mental alertness. The patient may refuse such drugs whether in the terminal stage or not and staff should not become impatient at such a refusal. The patient's wishes are to be respected. Buddhists usually maintain a strong acceptance of death and experience a peacefulness at death.

Handling of the deceased body

No formal or ritualistic functions are prescribed for the body. If a monk is present then (depending upon the school of Buddhism) many recite prayers for about one hour. The prayers do not have to be recited in the presence of the body. Therefore it is helpful for the relatives if a monk is informed as soon as possible after the death. The monk should be of the same school or tradition and background if possible.

Normal hospital procedure in preparation of the body after death is acceptable.

A Buddhist prefers cremation and that final disposal takes place between three and seven days after death.

Where Buddhist rites cannot be observed, any person may conduct the final service. There should be no reference to god, prayers, or doctrines of other religions. A memorial eulogy is accepted practice and a few passages from a Buddhist scripture may be read, if possible. If a Christian minister or priest is requested to conduct such a service, this should be considered seriously of course and she or he well prepared.

8. Bahá'í Faith

The Bahá'í faith is the newest of the major independent religions of the world. It originated in Iran in the mid-nineteenth century. The founder was the prophet Bahá'u'llah, which means "Glory to God".

The spread of this faith has been rather rapid. In 1984 it was reported as having over 112 000 centres and over 130 national bodies and five years later the report added at least another 70 to the list of countries. Its followers come from almost every cultural, social, racial and religious background.

The prophet had a chequered history, experiencing much persecution throughout his ministry. He was exiled to Akka (in modern Israel) where he died in 1892. He believed in God's progressive revelation to humankind himself before the latest of the prophets.

Bahá'í is an independent religion having its own laws and ordinances. It cannot be said to be a sect, or reform movement of any other religion or philosophical system. Unity, concord and harmony remain the core of its philosophy. The unit of God and his prophets and the human race is basic to Bahá'ism, so it encompasses and accepts most religions. This belief in the value of life and equality within life leads to the promotion of equal opportunities for all; the respect for life stresses universal peace. Religion and science are also inseparable; through this union a peaceful, ordered and progressive community is possible.

Each person possesses a soul which moves into another life after death. Cultivation of this soul is possible through obligatory daily prayer and scripture readings each morning and evening. Bahá'í belief in the immortality of the soul generates a confidence that there will be a new and greater life in the hereafter.

DIET AND FASTING

Bahá'í followers do not subscribe to any special dietary laws. Some may be vegetarians, though this is not a religious requirement. Bahá'ís do not drink alcohol except under medical direction.

Bahá'ís between the ages of 15 and 70 are expected to fast between sunrise and sunset from the 2nd March to 21st March each year. However fasting is not compulsory during hospitalisation, any illness, pregnancy, menstruation or when breast feeding.

RITUALS

There are no special religious requirements in cases of crisis. Birth is considered to be a happy occasion. Personal preference dictates the presence or otherwise of the husband at the time of delivery.

Ablutions and toilet practices demand no special requirements.

CARE OF THE ILL AND DYING

There is no priesthood and no sacramental requirements in the nursing or medical care of the sick. Therefore religious or pastoral care is of an entirely personal nature and is offered by religious friends or close relatives. The Bahá'í writings contain many prayers and meditations for spiritual and physical healing. These offer comfort and guidance to the patient and to relatives and friends.

Handling of the deceased body

There are no specific religious rituals prior to or following death. Normal nursing procedures are acceptable. A deceased Bahá'í may be wearing an inscribed ring, usually on the third or fourth finger of the right hand. This should not be buried with the body. The ring and any Bahá'í books should be kept aside and given into the care of Bahá'í relatives or members of the Bahá'í community. The handing over of these things to a Bahá'í is important if the deceased's relatives do not share the faith.

Under normal circumstances cremation is not allowed. The body must be buried within one hour's distance of the place of death. The burial service consists of Bahá'í prayers and readings from sacred texts. Recognised funeral directors may be used.

AUTOPSIES, TRANSFUSIONS, TRANSPLANTS

These are acceptable if performed on sound medical advice.

An autopsy is acceptable as long as the body is treated and returned with dignity.

A Bahá'í may leave his or her body for medical research on the proviso that the body is buried with dignity and not cremated or otherwise disposed of.

Organ donations are equally acceptable on similar conditions, that dignity is maintained. The donation of organs is in line with Bahá'í philosophy of helping other people and of ensuring harmony in the world.

ABORTION AND FAMILY PLANNING

The soul comes into being at conception. Abortion is therefore strongly discouraged, except for legitimate medical reasons, on the advice of a physician or preferably a panel of doctors.

Contraception presents no conflict for the Bahá'í. However, in vitro-fertilisation or other artificial means of conception are considered improper.

MODESTY

Bahá'ís generally have no preference for female or male health care professionals during their hospitalisation. Their belief in the unity of science and religion gives them a great respect for medical personnel and medical advice which leads to a belief that prescribed medications and prayer combine in the healing process.

9. Japanese beliefs and practices

For many in the Western world little is known of these people who, prior to World War II, remained largely within their own country and restricted entry by Westerners. Since its rapid economic growth and expansion, Japan is now a recognised world influence. Most people in Western countries are meeting Japanese people for the first time these days. They are welcomed as tourists and commercial investors.

There is still a basic ignorance of the Japanese and their culture, but the increasing possibility of Japanese people being admitted to our hospitals requires that some of that ignorance be overcome. However, the scope of this section only permits a very brief glimpse into the culture of the Japanese.

RELIGION IN JAPAN

When speaking of religion in Japan, we are thinking of many varieties. There is evidence that the Japanese are a very religious people. This was certainly the case up to World War II. The defeat of the Japanese in that war had repercussions upon the religion of the Emperor, whose family claims direct descent from the Sun Goddess, Amaterasu. That the God-Emperor Hirohito could be defeated shook much religious belief. The post-war industrial development of Japan seems to have weakened the structure of the society on which religion largely depended. The practice of religion in Japan today is a minority pursuit; a recent survey shows 30-35% of adults with religious affiliations, yet 70% believe that religious sentiment is important.

The indigenous religion of Japan is Shintoism. This has been part of Japanese life for some two thousand years. Confucianism, which came to Japan via Korea during the sixth century AD, has often been considered more of a philosophy, with moral and ethical precepts, than a religion. About the same time Buddhism was introduced from China and rapidly gained royal patronage.

St. Francis Xavier introduced Christianity to Japan in 1549. It spread and grew quite rapidly; but the current Christian population is less than one per cent.

The common people have amalgamated many religious practices to form syncretic folk religions, known as "new religious movements", some of which were established earlier, but only gained official recognition after 1949.

The new religions appeal to the people who are lost in the concrete jungles of urban living. They are strong in magical practice, with an emphasis on relevant issues such as family and health, and are not concerned with the religious questions on the future life.

In this section, Shintoism and Japanese Buddhism will be expanded to further Westerner understanding of their beliefs and practices.

SHINTOISM

The name Shinto goes back to prehistoric times. The religion has undergone much transformation from its earliest beginnings and has affected the socio-cultural life of Japan's people. Even in the twentieth century, its political ramifications echoed around the world during World War II.

Currently it may be considered under four main forms: Shinto of the imperial house; shrine Shinto; sect Shinto and folk Shinto.

Shinto of the imperial house
This form involved the rites and worship of imperial ancestors and is observed at special royal family shrines. The Emperor usually officiates at these ceremonies, to which rites the general public are not admitted. Its fate in Japan suffered as a result of World War II and Emperor Hirohito's "abdicating" his divine powers in 1945. On this basis the new constitution of Japan was adopted.

From the Meija era of the mid-nineteenth century, state Shinto developed as a combination of Shinto of the imperial house and shrine Shinto. State Shinto became a government institution, with the priests as government servants. This remained the case until the end of World War II.

Shrine Shinto

Shrine Shinto was separated from the state in February, 1946, becoming a purely religious body. The main principles of shrine Shinto are:

- To be grateful for the blessings of the Kami (the divine beings of heaven and earth) and the blessings of the ancestors, and to be diligent in the observance of Shinto rituals, applying oneself to them with sincerity, cheerfulness and purity of heart;

- to be helpful to others in the world at large through deeds of service, without thought of reward, and to seek the advancement of the world as one whose life mediates the will of the Kami;

- to bind oneself with others in harmonious acknowledgement of the will of the Emperor, praying that the country may flourish and that other peoples too may live in peace and prosperity.

The shrine built as places of worship are to be plain in design and material, characterised by simplicity, purity and harmony. They house ashes and relics of the dead, store works of art, and are the dwelling places of the Kami.

Rituals, principally are for purification, namely:

- *Rites of preliminary purification:* this involves the avoiding of all foods (except those prepared over a ritually pure fire) and the total immersion of the body in the sea or river: certain taboos concerning recently-bereaved persons and menstruating women are observed.

- *Rites of internal purification:* the priest, using a wand, symbolically cleanses the object or worshippers to be purified.
- *Rites of dedication:* originating from harvest festival rituals, sprigs of the sacred sakaki tree, rice, sake, etc. are offered. The prayers offering praise to the Kami, intercessions for blessing, personal dedication and pledges of right loving complete the service.

Successive generations are represented in the Kami, which places value on ancestors and the importance of future generations.

Sect Shinto

The promulgation of freedom of religion in Japan in 1889 created a problem for the government: the thirteen religious groups which sprang up between 1876 and 1908 were typical of Shinto forms, but the state was loathe to absorb them into Shrine Shinto, so sect Shinto which would embrace these groups was adopted. Like the post-war new religions, Sect Shinto emphasised contemporary life in contrast with stress upon any future life.

Folk Shinto

Folk Shinto is a primitive kind of Shintoism which is a mixture of superstition, magic-religious rites, kinship ties and practices of the common people.

BUDDHISM

Buddhism was introduced into Japan about 538 AD, an early convert being Prince Shotoku about the year 600, who saw Buddhism as a means of attaining his two goals:

- to establish a single central government under the authority of the emperor thus unifying the various clans;
- to raise the cultural level of Japan.

Even at this period there were desires to keep Japanese values intact and to adapt Buddhism to fit these. A century later temples were being built with government subsidies. Some major developments of Buddhism took place:

- Appearing from China whose culture was seen to be more advanced, the Japanese imperial family and the aristocracy embraced Buddhism, so it moved from the aristocracy downwards.
- The patronage of the Emperor resulted in a strong bond between Buddhism and the state. This relationship is significantly unique. Every citizen has to register at a particular temple for instance.
- Buddhism adapted itself into the family life of Japan with a strong emphasis on ancestor worship and holding services for the dead.

FOLK RELIGION

Folk religion may include worship at family Shinto or Buddhist shrines as well as at village sites to honour the particular Kami. Ancestors are worshipped for their support in the practical things of life: the future, illness and similar matters. Weddings are usually performed according to Shinto tradition, whilst funerals are the prerogative of the Buddhist priests.

Many of the newer religions in Japan, such as sect Shinto, are traceable back to folk religion; the influence of folk religion stretches across all strata of society from urban to non-urban, the affluent to the poor.

NAMES

According to Japanese convention the family name comes first, then the given name. Some Japanese travellers and those who are living in Western countries are following the Western practice of putting the given name first, then the family name. It would be prudent to establish which is the family name to maintain true medical records and identification.

CARE OF THE ILL AND DYING

Informing patients and relatives of diagnosis

If the illness is non-terminal (nor life-threatening) then the doctor may inform the patient and family of all the facts. Many Japanese doctors do not tell their patients and patients do not ask.

Japanese culture involves subtle innuendo where the condition is terminal. Doctors hesitate to give any diagnosis and prognosis; they merely say that more tests are needed which may require prolonged hospitalisation. Where the condition has exhausted treatment possibilities, the specialist will suggest the patient may go home, indicating that the patient may go home to die in comfort and peace with the family. The family usually know the truth, though

Japanese people tend to believe that the patient may not be emotionally capable of handling the true diagnosis. The family then accept the responsibility to emotionally support and comfort the terminal patient.

LENGTH OF HOSPITALISATION

Japanese expect to spend longer periods in hospital than is the case generally in the West. For a minor operation a week to ten days is normal, whilst for major surgery, it may be a month or more. This is partly due to health insurance schemes, where the longer the stay, the cheaper it becomes. There are three types:
- National insurance where government pays approx. 70%;
- Company insurance where company pays approx. 90%;
- Worker's compensation where insurance pays approx. 60%.

The length of stay in hospital should be explained so that a Japanese patient does not consider the treatment is not as adequate or good as in Japan.

DIET AND FASTING

Rice is the staple food of Japan, with very little spicy or fried content. Western hospital food is normally acceptable. The Japanese eat a rice gruel (*ôkayu*) when convalescing. (It is a simple one measure of rice to two of water slowly boiled until tender and soft, a little salt added during the cooking.) Ôkayu

JAPANESE BELIEFS AND PRACTICES 83

may be offered to the patient as the Japanese are
reticent about making direct requests.

PASTORAL AND SPIRITUAL CARE

In Japanese Buddhism, prayer is important for personal benefits. In the Western world, the possibility
of a Shinto or Japanese Buddhist priest being available is unlikely. A Japanese patient would not
expect any form of pastoral or spiritual care, but the
hospital chaplain may be able to provide spiritual
support and be a religious presence to the patient. A
short prayer by the chaplain using the name of God
rather than Jesus would generally be accepted.

Should a suitable Buddhist priest or nun be available, it is, of course advisable to seek the patient's
permission to call him or her.

AUTOPSIES, TRANSFUSIONS,
TRANSPLANTS

Japan is keen to catch up in the transplant field of
medicine, though traditional ethics have largely
been against transplants.

Live donor transplants of kidneys in Japan have
taken place, although medical ethnics committees
are still debating the matter. Thus questions of
transplants and organ donation at this stage would
probably receive a negative response, although
some Japanese opt for overseas transplant opera-
tions to avoid the Japanese bans and indecision.

Transfusions produce a clouded response, the
AIDS situation may be a deterrent. A fear for the

Japanese in a hospital outside Japan is that "foreign" blood may be contaminated, thus creating a reluctance to accept a transfusion. Ascertain from relatives or patient the attitude to transfusions.

Autopsies for coroner's courts or to ascertain exact cause of death are generally accepted. If a Japanese tourist should die, there is a possibility that an autopsy would be necessary if there is little previous medical history available.

ABLUTIONS

In Japan, the Japanese use Asian-type toilet facilities, that is, they require water for toilet cleansing purposes. In the West, they adapt readily to Western bathroom fixtures, most are comfortable using toilet paper. However there may be a few who need water to be made available. Water for washing hands before meals is another requirement.

MODESTY

Japanese women generally are very modest in matters concerning their body. They prefer to be treated by a nurse or doctor of the same sex. However, they recognise the professionalism of hospital personnel and are willing to waive this preference. Particular efforts should be made by male health workers to respect the dignity of Japanese women in their care.

Handling the deceased body
All jewellery is to be removed and returned to family. Where family or priest's counsel is unavailable,

normal hospital procedure will be acceptable to the Japanese, who will later follow their own customs.

The Japanese would not expect foreigners to prepare a patient in Buddhist style; this becomes a family responsibility. Where the family is unavailable, a Buddhist priest should be notified if possible. The deceased is dressed in a white kimono and wears straw shoes called *waraji*. The ceremonial clothing is called *shiro shozoku*.

Appendix

RELIGIOUS FOOD OBSERVANCE

The observance of food law is an important part of some traditions. To break a food law would be unthinkable, some would be physically repulsed. Guilt, disgust, shame and even illness sometimes ensue when even inadvertently one of these laws is infringed.

Westernisation has weakened the resolve of many to maintain religious food prescriptions. Patients' dietary needs should be part of the questionnaire at the time of hospital admission so that the patient's requirements can be accommodated.

GUIDELINES:
PERMITTED AND PROHIBITED FOODS

	Hindus Buddhists	Sikhs	Muslims	Jews
Eggs	some*	yes	yes	yes
Milk and yoghurt	yes	yes	yes	yes
Cottage/curd cheese	yes	yes	yes	yes
Chicken	some*	some	halal+	kosher++
Mutton	some*	some	halal+	kosher++
Beef	no	no	halal+	kosher++
Pork	no	rarely	no	no
Fish	some*	some	yes	yes
Butter/ghee	yes	yes	yes	yes
Margarine/ vegetable oils	yes	yes	yes	yes

* Very strict followers avoid this.
+ Halal meat must be killed, dedicated and prepared in a special way.
++Kosher meat for Jews requires special rituals and
  butchering procedures in preparation.

References

Agency for Cultural Affairs *Japanese Religion: a Survey* (Tokyo: Kodansha) 7th edition 1989

Carmody, D. L. and Carmody, J. T. *Prayer in World Religions* (Maryknoll, N.Y:Orbis) 1990

Hospital Chaplaincies Council *Our Ministry and Other Faiths* (London: C 10 Publications) 1983

Kirkwood N. A. "Caring for Arabic Muslims Experiencing Hospitalisation in Australia" unpublished dissertation (San Francisco Theological Seminary) 1986

Lothian Community Relations Council *Religious and Cultures* (Edinburgh, U.K.) 1984

Neuberger, J. *Caring for Dying People of Different Faiths* (London: Austen Cornish Publishers) 1987

Nursing Times "Death with Dignity" series, Vol. 85, (London) 1989